Fire Mobile

(the pregnancy sonnets)

also available
by Matthew Porubsky

voyeur poems
Coal City Press
mppoetry.com

other titles from Woodley Press

Begin Again: 150 Kansas Poems
    edited by Caryn Mirriam-Goldberg
Sky Land
    Michael Johnson
Kansas Poems
    William Stafford edited by Denise Low
Ghost Stories of the New West:
From Einstein's Brain to Geromino's Boots
    Denise Low
Finding the Edge
    Al Ortolani
Lisa's Flying Electric Piano
    Kevin Rabas
From the Inisde Out
    Brian Daldorph
Certain Dawn, Inevitable Dawn
    Tasha Haas
Atlas of Our Birth
    Serina Allison Hearn
Fugitive Histories
    Harley Elliott
Sould's Night Out
    Nedra Rogers
Standing on the Edge of the World
    Lindsay Martin-Bowen

washburn.edu/reference/woodley-press/

Fire Mobile
(the pregnancy sonnets)

by Matthew Porubsky

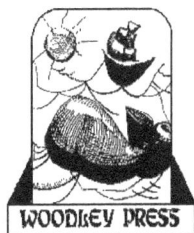

WOODLEY PRESS

Edited by Dennis Etzel Jr.

Printed by Lightning Source
Cover art: Stella Robbins
Cover and book design: Leah Sewell

Woodley Press
Department of English
Washburn University
Topeka, KS 66621
washburn.edu/reference/woodley-press/index.html

ISBN: 978-0-9828752-4-7

Several poems in this collection have been published in the
following journals: *I-70 Review, Inscape, freefall, Coal City Review, The
Journal* (UK,) *Little Balkans Review, RowHouse Poetry Revue, Blue Island
Review* and *seveneightfive magazine.* I would like to thank the editors
for their support.

Thanks to Leah Sewell, Dennis Etzel Jr., Kevin Rabas, Brian
Daldorph, Thomas Fox Averill, Eric McHenry, Caryn Mirriam-
Goldberg, Ande Davis, Stella Robbins, Daniel Billen, Bailey and
Justin Marable, Melissa Sewell, Brie Martin, Zach Johnsrud and Dr.
Jennifer Harader for reading this manuscript and sharing ideas.

Thanks to Manya Schmidt CNM, for her guidance and care.

Thanks to the musical inspiration of Björk's "Vespertine"
and Julie Doiron's "Goodnight Nobody."

Special thanks to Stella Robbins for the incredible artwork.
And Leah Sewell for all kinds of creating.

mppoetry.com
mmporubsky@gmail.com

for

Leah, Sylvia, Oliver

Mom and Dad

Introduction

by Dennis Etzel Jr.

When Matthew Porubsky gave me an earlier version of *Fire Mobile* to read, I could not foresee that I would be handed this version years later to publish through Woodley Press.

"How would you pronounce the title?" Matt first asked.

"Fire Mo-beel," I said, with the long e sound for "mobile," as in automobile. I realized "mobile" could also be pronounced "mo-bill"—the way people pronounce it often as an adjective, as something movable.

It's a wonderful double entendre for describing a pregnancy—as a fire that is both movable and in motion, circling above, to captivate a baby's attention. With a poet's attention, these sonnets are records of the nine-month travel, honest and revealing. Matt writes to capture the joys and frustrations of being a mother-to-be, like in "(The Idea Alone)" in the second section, describing how people assume they can go up to touch someone's belly when they are pregnant:

> *"I humor them, but that's so personal.*
> *They're stealing from me like some casual*
> *shoplifter." Your hand slides a guarding path*
> *down your cradle as you envision scenes*
> *of protecting your child by any means.*

Along with the poems are mini-introductions for each section, descriptions of each trimester. With subjects like dreams, the body, family, and the writer reflecting on the beloved sleeping, this collection captures pregnancy via different lenses.

Matt finds the best form for conveying this through the sonnet and its different forms, including Shakespearean and Petrarchan. Aside from the rule of fourteen lines, ten syllables to a line, and the different rhyme schemes based on what kind of sonnet is used, the sonnet has its history of having a *volta*, a turn at the eighth line, moving from conflict to resolution, or showing a contrast of things. Another part of the sonnet's history is of its poet addressing the Beloved, as this collection does.

These poems are the intimate moments between mother and father. However, I also enjoy the touches of humor, like in a poem about the different kinds of foods that should be eaten, and avoided: "These whirled warnings ax / your mind until you are nearly queasy / while all you want are eggs over-easy" "(Restrictions, Etc.)." This is another aspect about this collection that is wonderful: the lack of sentimentality. One could easily dive into sentimental waters when writing poems about such a subject as pregnancy, but Matt travels the range of authenticity throughout his tribute.

Likewise, there are dashes of the mystery. Meditating on the overall journey, where a woman's body transforms to do what needs to be done at each moment throughout the pregnancy, there are moments when Matt writes a tribute to the sacred mother—via the mother-union with The Goddess Mother:

> You pull me to you and my body slips
> between yours, sighing blessed and hallow.
> Then truly begins the adoration –
> you, an image of ancient creation. "(Idol Worship)"

"The breath" can be found throughout this book—one of the most interesting aspects to me as someone who loves poetry. In the third "(The Idea)," the mother makes an exclamation: "'It moves with me…with my breathing…with my belly.'" There is a poetic idea about the breath, too, as Li-Young Lee said the breath determines utterance and often lasts for ten syllables. As Lee refers to this like each line in a sonnet, we might draw a parallel here: how the mother is making a connection to her child through breathing, how the poet makes a connection with tradition through the sonnet form. If poetry asks for a deeper attention in its writing, with the awareness of the soon-to-be-mother, the poet of these sonnets privileges poem, mother, and yet-to-be-born equally. As sonnets have a history of being written to a Beloved, the mother becomes that Beloved—the Mother-Becoming. I am thankful to watch this book's release into the world.

Dennis Etzel Jr.
May 2011

Contents

Prologue

- The Fervor   17

    Detail One   19

First Trimester: Realization Day

- (To a Mother Soon, Sleeping)   23
- (First Dream)   24
- (Quick-Steadied Footing)   25
- (Weighing One Ounce)   27
- (Passively Outfitting the Room)   28
- (Idol Worship)   29
- (Second Dream – A Nap)   30
- (Quick Change)   31
- (Restrictions, Etc.)   32
- (The Book)   33
- (The Idea Itself)   34
- (Third Dream)   36

    Detail Two   39

Second Trimester: Maturation Day

- (To a Mother Soon, Sleeping)   43
- (Fourth Dream)   45
- (One Pound a Week)   46
- (Between Breaths)   47
- (Olfactory Upgrade)   48
- (Concerns, Etc.)   49
- (Subtle Construction)   51
- (Bath Tub Message)   52
- (The Idea Alone)   53
- (Idol Worship)   54
- (Fifth Dream)   56
- (Stretching Wakeup)   57

Detail Three   59

Third Trimester : Preparation Day

- (To a Mother Soon, Sleeping)   63
- (Sixth Dream)   65
- (The Lightening)   66
- (Weight, Etc.)   67
- (A Number of Games)   68
- (Seventh Dream – A Nap)   69
- (Tectonic Movements)   70
- (The Skeleton Inside)   72
- (The Idea)   73
- (Idol Worship)   75
- (Eighth Dream)   76
- (Ready)   77

Epilogue

- Falling Action   81

Fire Mobile
(the pregnancy sonnets)

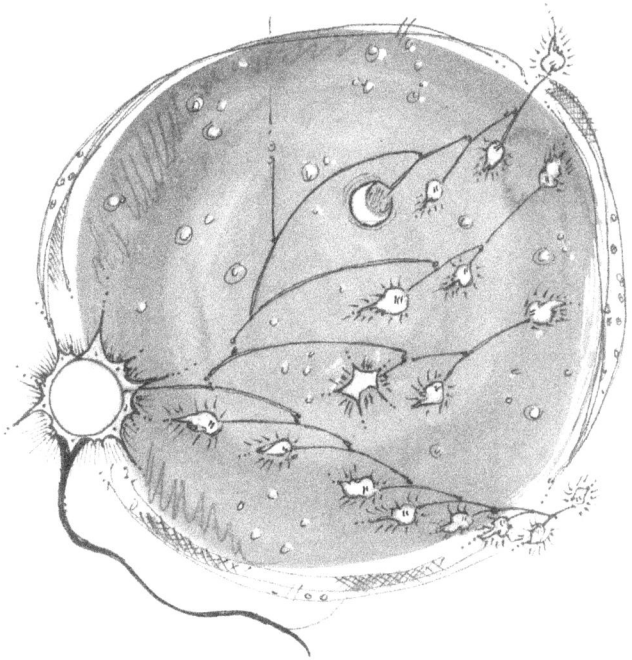

Prologue

The Fervor

Flirting into the barriers around
flesh in a grading trance unrelenting,
the stumble of each move is tightly wound
as momentum. It steers complementing

segments, flaring hot and mute, to surface
in random waves unsteady. The dim course
is a slit to us – a condensed preface
unfolding and surrounding a moist source

of sectioned overlays. Blindly we swerve,
hinged in loose clasps and grips, to lilting sighs
that follow the cantor of skin and nerves.
There is no great awareness of the sly

slip of the cell unconsciously imposed –
only melded forms collapsing enclosed.

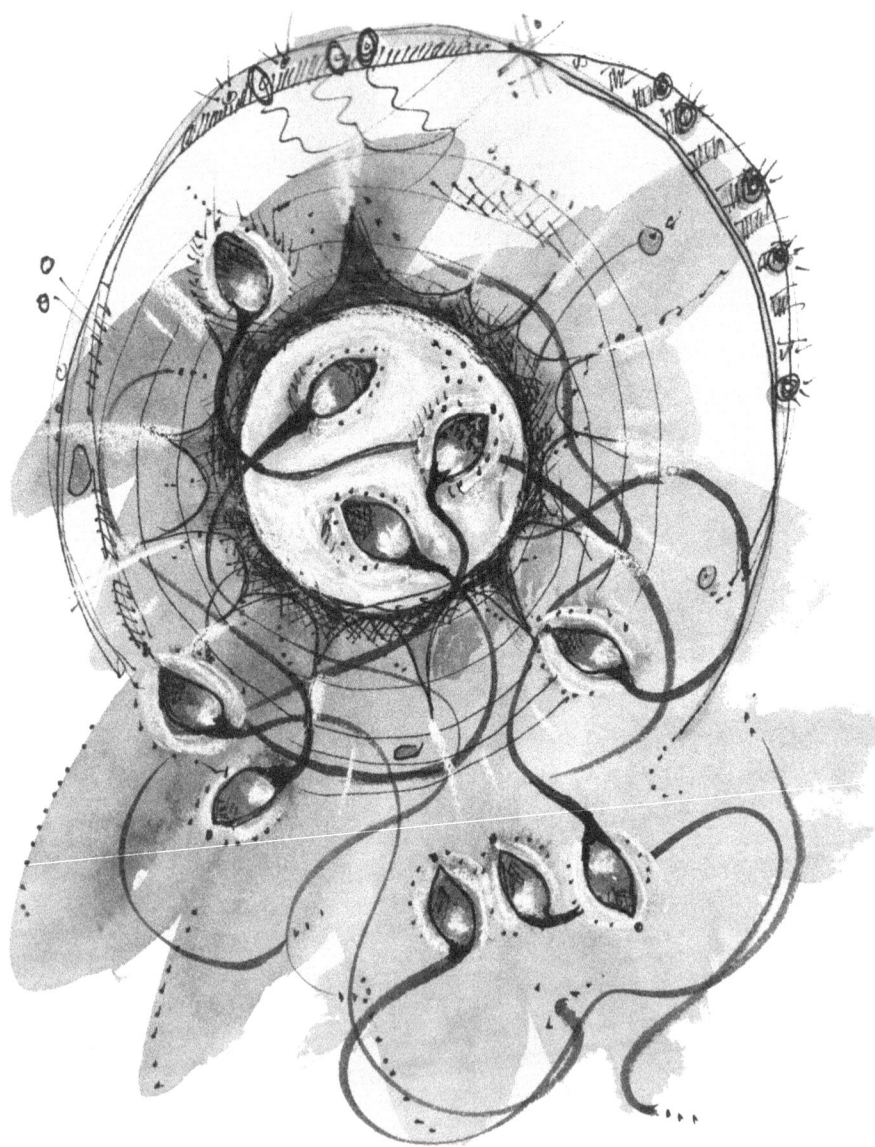

Detail One

The first twelve weeks of pregnancy are relatively secretive. The mother shows little weight gain and the conceived only weighs up to an ounce and measures about three inches by the end of the trimester; the size of a plum. This time is usually filled with preoccupations and apprehensions about the coming change of lifestyle.

The pregnancy may show itself in symptoms such as breast growth and tenderness, visible blue veins beneath the breasts and abdomen, nausea coupled with vomiting, dizziness, headaches, food cravings and aversions, mood swings, and fatigue. The mother may also have startling and strange dreams that persist throughout the remainder of the pregnancy.

The conceived develops inside a sac of fluids where it grows protected.

First Trimester :
Realization Day

(To a Mother Soon, Sleeping)

Sometimes I can hear the grit of your teeth
in the middle of the night, the simple
moan when your forehead rests on my temple.
You lick your lips, searching for taste beneath,

a leftover love of the smoke they've years
entertained, missing the subtle, soft curl
it twinged at their sides – a smile to unfurl
slowly where you could hide or disappear.

Now, you're left with breaths of plain air heated
by you and the new fire mobile, spinning
hard and low in your belly, beginning
to learn of balance until completed

and absolute. Still sleeping, your fingers,
where pleasure was held, tap where it lingers.

(First Dream)

There is a city here. Tousled unknowns
fill each space, each inch within the shadow
of unmentioned streets and alleys below
lonely skyscrapers and tenements. Down

overcast avenues, graffiti crowns
walls randomly, written in high and low
arches and crossings. There are no fellow
dreamers here in your solitary town.

You walk the chipped bricks, a smoke in one hand
and a drink in the other, humming tunes
of possibilities and passions found

newly stale. With the final sip, this land
sheds to paper, crumpled and bent. These ruins
ignite from your flicked smoke in flames unbound.

(Quick-Steadied Footing)

You shimmy off the sea-salt of sleeping,
unconscious waves of your heartbeats and dreams,
one hand below the cloud slowly building
in your belly which stretches to its seams

daily. Off-balanced steps center part-way
across the veneer, steadied by your breath,
as you envision the plotline in play
that changes your aplomb by length and breadth.

This embodied growth is partnered throughout -
swift draped hair on your shoulders, nails in quick
reaching, blouse unbuttoning. This about
you is a building, a timpani wick

lit and burning the shine of small kindling
to glow as a drumming never dwindling.

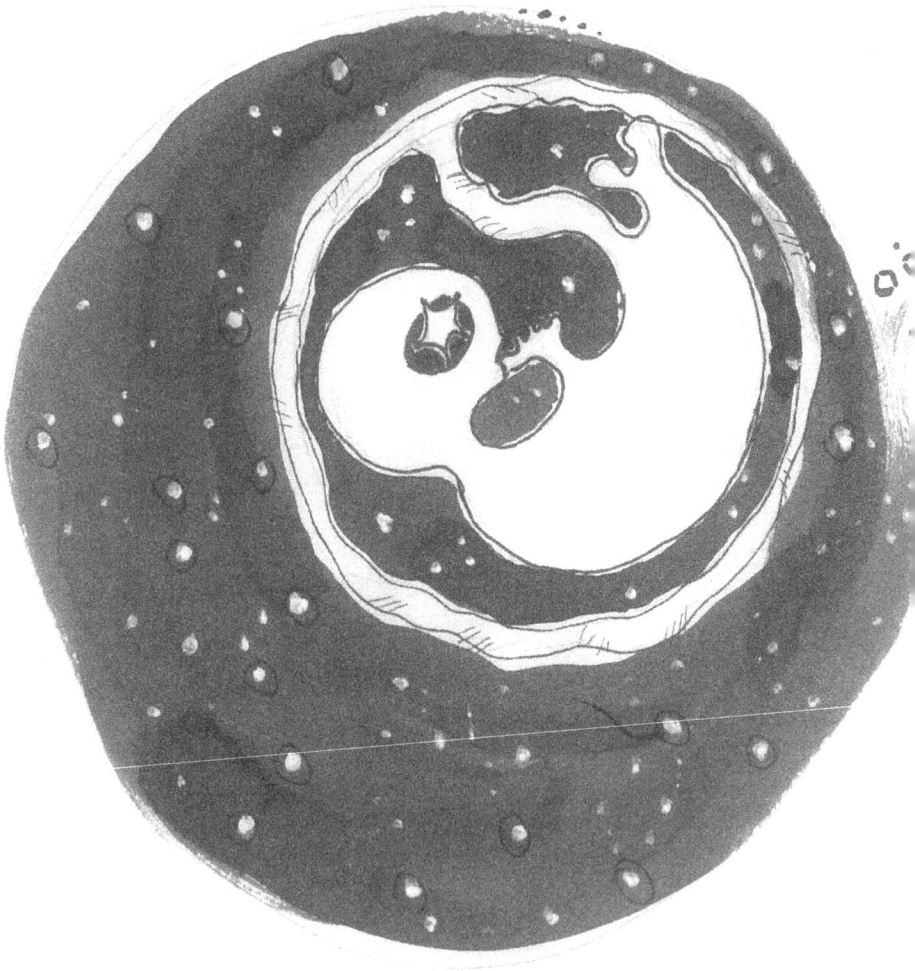

(Weighing One Ounce)

It seems an intangible abstract now,
like a step off a cliff, an arm asleep
as blood returns to the veins' steady creep,
the watery shadow of old window

pane glass. If there were a window to see
inside, perhaps it would be more defined,
less rehearsed words to hide ideas behind,
a picture other than what might just be

more tummy reflected in the mirror.
This view would rearrange reasons, give sight
to feeling, proof to the sickness, delight
to pains. Underneath this tiny parlor

you could measure its fit in your cupped hand
exact, line to line, where head and feet land.

(Passively Outfitting the Room)

You've kept the baby's room quite bare, afraid
that you may jinx the whole thing, but you smiled,
taking the knitted sweater your aunt made
along with a white changing table piled

with wipes and lotions. You gladly received
a sock monkey from my mother inside
the family crib and you hardly believed
my sister's early present as you eyed

the white onesie holding its shoulders by
fingertips in front of you, first seeing
the image to come and fill that you ply
fixed within. You put these in drawers, being

nervous to stare, and leave the room's door closed,
for now keeping the mystery unclothed.

(Idol Worship)

This vision of you heightens the moment.
The sheets hardly hide your newness fleshing.
Slowly, my hand starts its praising movement
at the deep of your thigh, close to meshing

hair curling moist, and rises at the hill
of your stomach's soft distention. Shallow
veins underlay my path, each moment still
and shuttering to shine your skin halo

bright. Your breasts lie wide, mimicking your hips'
crescents, overlapping in thin shadows.
You pull me to you and my body slips
between yours, sighing blessed and hallow.

Then truly begins the adoration –
you, an image of ancient creation.

(Second Dream – A Nap)

The sky is lit limitless, glowing gray
from the landscaped snow fallen and falling
feathered. You're bundled close with down filling,
hooded and zipped to warmth. Some steps away,

in the piling whiteness, a baby lies
naked. Your steps slide to see its bawling
wet face, but no sound is made. The sprawling
blank scene is silent except for the sighs

of your breathing. Kneeling, you try to scoop
the soundless weeping newborn in your arms,
only to push it deeper in the snow.

Rapidly sweeping off the snow, you stoop
low, hoping that your breath will somehow warm
the quiet writhing as blood freezes slow.

(Quick Change)

It is sudden. Fast as lighting a match
but silent and without the flint signal,
this irrational chemical tendril
constricts your mood whole. Helplessly I watch

you ride this swing in playground style, clenching
the chains in tight fists. Barely in the clear
of your rise and fall, I maneuver near
your emotional edge, frailly flinching

as I'm tangled unintentionally.
Your tone and slant glare strike with sudden speed
and stall short seconds before you proceed
to place the next bite but, casually,

you wink gently and walk away changing,
tension and flirtation rearranging.

(Restrictions, Etc.)

This list keeps growing longer every day:
you battle with caffeine limitations,
dodging the aroma invitations
of coffee and green tea, you try to stay

away from hotdogs, lunch meat and raw sprouts
to the dismay of your random cravings,
they suggest fish oil capsules for staving
off seafood's chance of mercury, count out

heated blankets and hot tubs to relax,
be sure your bug repellent has no deet,
avoid lifting heavy objects, retreat
from secondhand smoke. These whirled warnings tax

your mind until you are nearly queasy
while all you want are eggs over-easy.

(The Book)

"I hate this damn cover," you say, tossing
the book to the floor, sliding from upright
to lying in bed. The woman of spite
reads the same book on the front, eyes glossing

with somber preparation and patience.
This thick guide of complete information
outlines the aspects of expectation
and plants grief with relief. The occurrence

of your details in the mix starts breeding
simple apprehensions into brooding
preoccupations of worry flooding
your thoughts. You glare back, down at the reading

woman with her months-long belly. She rocks
unmoving with a glare and smug head-cock.

(The Idea Itself)

"My grandmother had similar symptoms
I have, at one point," you say as you hold
a pillow to your stomach. These customs
of construction are millennia old.

Your neck bends back along the top edge curve
of the striped sofa. "How more could any
one person affect the world than to have
a child?" Your eyes close – dream like so many.

The pillow falls to your thighs as your neck
tilts and you let loose your hair. Each strand lands
down the back of the sofa. "It's a speck
in the span of generations." Your hands

comb your hair up and back. Your thought-weary
eyes blink soft. "It seems so ordinary."

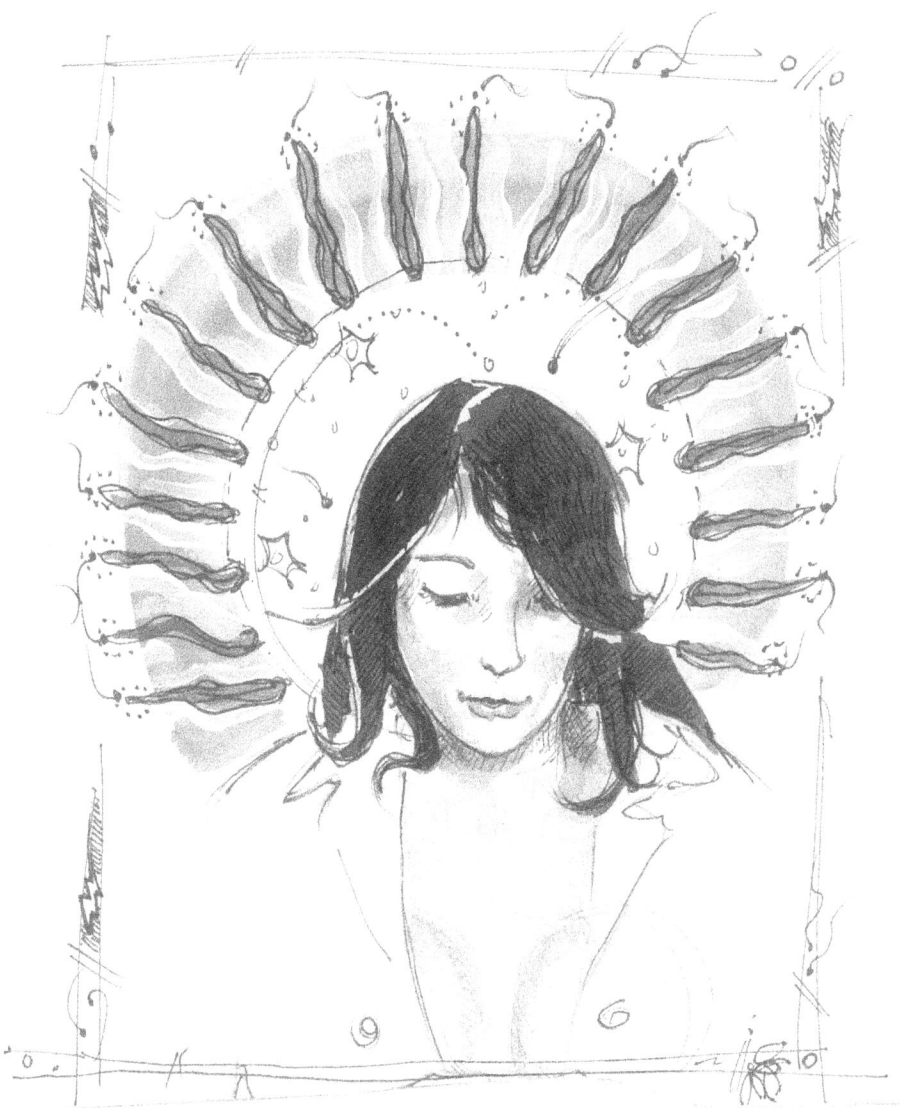

(Third Dream)

Your shallow stomach rapidly expands
as you watch. It swells straight forward, bending
to a rounded lobe, stiff and tight, sending
nerve shivering hums scattered as you stand

speechless of the speed. You don't understand,
gripping a hold against your distending
skin as it pauses – growth at its ending.
Then it's gone and your belly sinks as sand

inside of you. The child now sits ahead
of you, its naked, wrinkled skin glows flush.
Grass begins to grow along its eyebrows

and chin while leaves and petals tightly thread
slender floral braids across its skin, lush
and layered, hiding all beneath flowered rows.

Detail Two

The second trimester, lasting until the beginning of the seventh month, has the most prevalent physical upheaval of the three. The mother usually gains an average of one pound a week, while the conceived will grow to about fourteen inches and weigh in the area of a pound and a half. By the end of this trimester it is about the size of a bag of flour. Fatigue tends to drift away and the mother is reenergized with her adjusting and transforming body.

Skin at the abdomen and breasts may begin to itch, stretching further. The abdomen swells to near the rib cage, slowly compressing the lungs, while the nipples and areola widen, darkening in color. Back pain becomes frequent along with mild swelling of the feet and hands, a more demanding appetite, nasal congestion and nosebleeds, leg cramps, and the first appearance of stretch marks and varicose veins. Nausea usually fades but can be replaced by heartburn and indigestion from organs rearranging to accommodate the growing inside.

The conceived fully develops its heart and kidneys, as well as fingernails and eyebrows. The umbilical cord thickens in order to transport nourishment. Its sex can now be determined and it is capable of hearing the mother's and its own heartbeat. Other external sounds are muffled, but are also audible.

The mother will experience the first fetal movements. This is known as "the quickening."

Second Trimester :
Maturation Day

(To a Mother Soon, Sleeping)

You're asleep on your back with joints tightly
set unmoving. A week ago, you asked
me not to let you sleep this way, lightly
move you if you were so sleeping. Now, tasked

as your body's night watchman, I pay close
attention with closed eyes to your dark turns
and returns of uncomfortable pose
as you search between heavy sighs, concerns

of blood flow and aches as subconscious dreams.
Now, I see your leveled position found,
shoulders flat and neck stretched in ease. It seems
an innocent deviation around

your binding belly. I sidle beside
you and nudge just enough to say I tried.

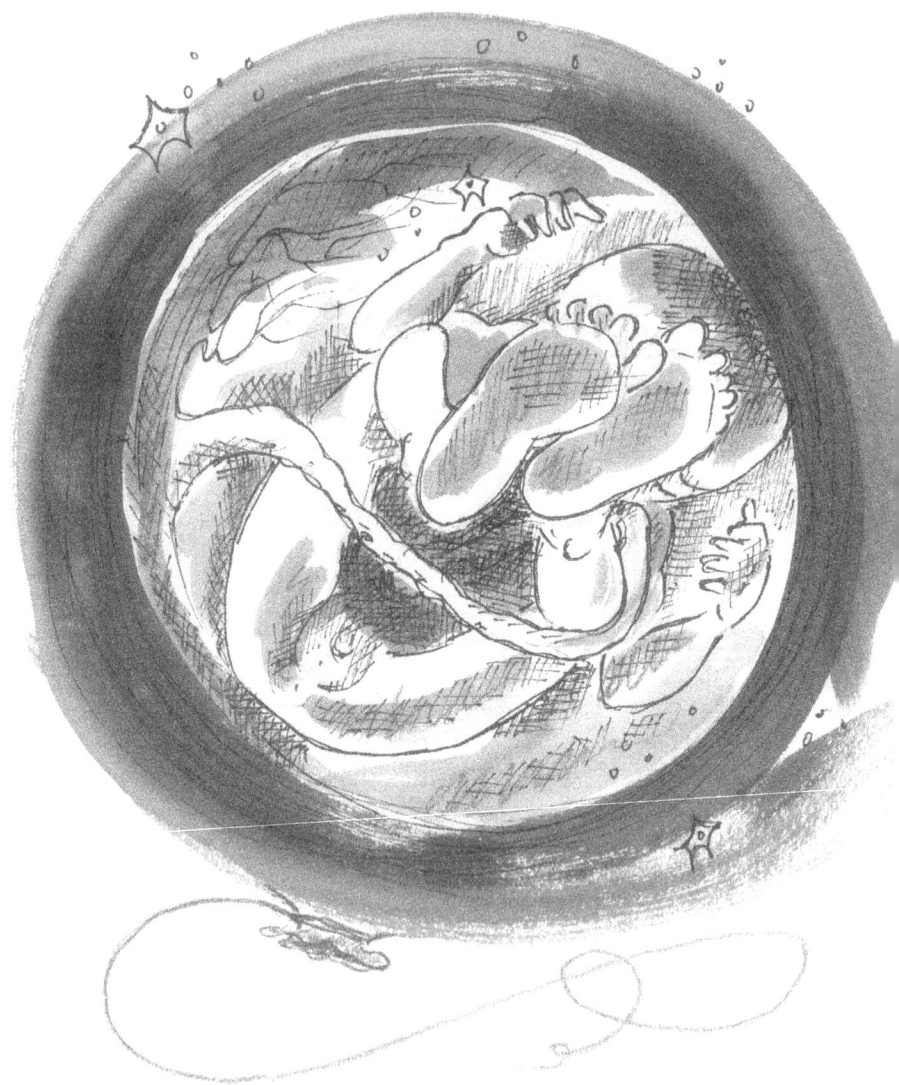

(Fourth Dream)

You can't tell if it's one or the other
as it floats, still as the air on all sides.
Its fetal hover turns but always hides
its sex. Anxiously you wait another

revolution, determining whether
or not you can instinctively decide
the solution based solely on how wide
the head is, how long the feet are – mother's

intuition in action. Then you reach,
determined to discover what's hiding
there in suspension, but your arms hold tight

at your waist. Stuck in their newly carved niche,
your useless arms fumble from the chiding
answer that spins secretly in plain sight.

(One Pound a Week)

You can't help but hear the whispered visions
from the mirror. This recent indulgence,
the way your eyes scroll your changed appearance,
possesses. You gasp in breathless motions,

soundless acknowledgments of your body
nude and new. Your skin stretches tight, from hips
to your shallowing navel. Each itch wisps
faintly for you to feel the slow broody

movement. A fresh crease shines unfolded just
above your stomach, between your spreading
breasts and the wings of your ribs. A dreading
of fullness lingers in your eyes like dust

on the mirror. You stand unsure, the weight
behind your skin clouding what you create.

(Between Breaths)

The clothes you pull from the dryer are still
warm and the house is quiet and settled
as you begin. A song softly distills
slow, sound fostering down to the huddle

of your stomach. "I'm going to love you
like nobody loves you, come rain or come
shine." You only sing between bends, breaths too
compressed and cut as you reach. It's become

a comfort, a song that will soothe faint whines
and cries when the baby has left your heart's
beat. "Happy together...won't it be fine."
Lifting piles of cooled folds, a rolling starts

in you – the movement of stretching confined.
"I'll love you always, baby, rain or shine."

(Olfactory Upgrade)

It seems your sense of smell has reached a new
level, somewhere near supernatural -
in the dumpster outside, there is a slew
of oranges that turned from the usual

citrus scent to the mustiness of rum,
the subtle warning of rain in the air
hours in advance, the spot on the rug from
the dog, cleaned and cleaned again, the soft flare

of open honeysuckle down the street,
the dust in every corner, steaming hot
tea now time travels you to the past, sweet
pea lotion is heaven on earth, and not

a day goes by when you don't sniff to say
there's a cigarette lit some miles away.

(Concerns, Etc.)

You can't help but imagine that you might
be doing it all wrong, that each instinct
needs to be rethought, that you're not in sync
with what is best for your child. Is a tight

cramp an early sign of impending doom
or indigestion? How frequently should
the baby move and what in the world could
happen if you slipped and fell? Is the room

going to be ready in time and how
long will labor last and if you'll survive,
if the baby will make it through alive?
Will it be healthy or will it soon know

your voice and that you've waited with tired eyes
to see which small features you recognize?

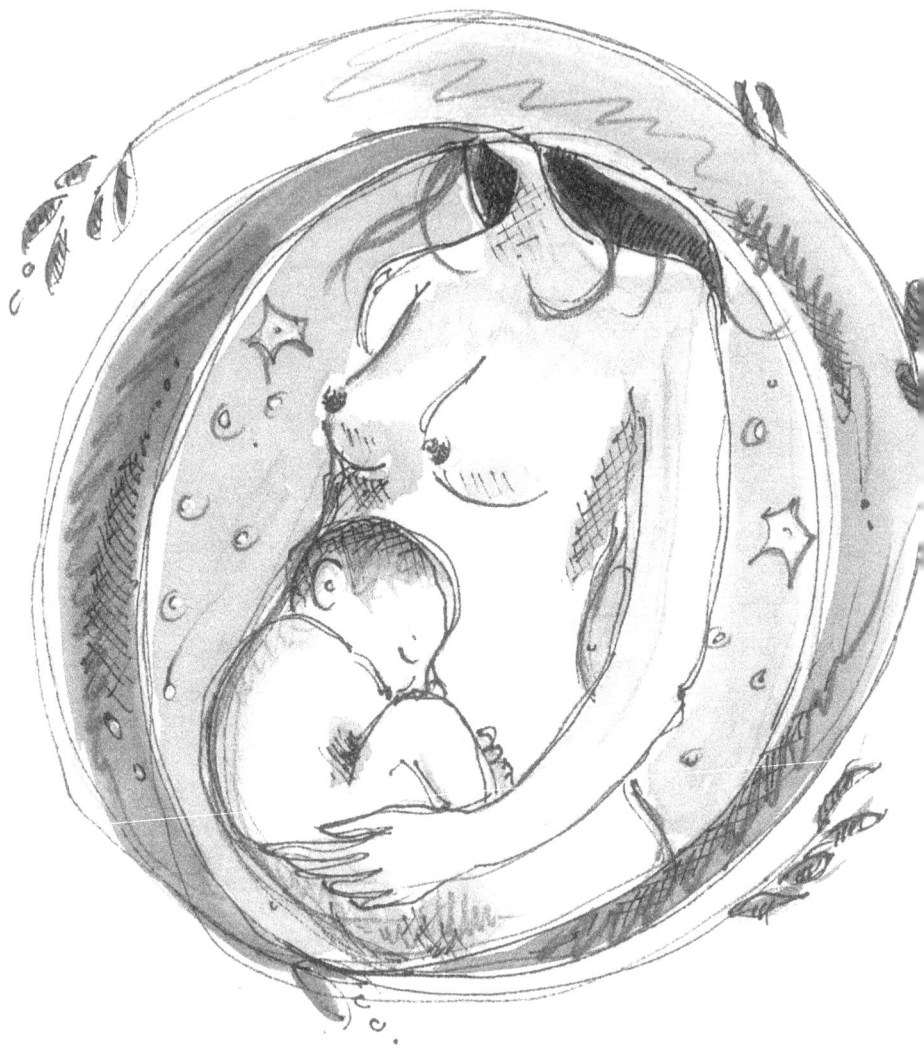

(Subtle Construction)

You don't bother to explain your techniques.
The unconscious system of translating
yourself to skin and bone, oscillating
mid-body, develops daily. Instincts

lead you to weave liquid to fingerprints,
folded and patterned, into a design
never imagined or matched. You refine
cells into eyelids and toenails of mint

condition, small silk spins of protection,
and filter sounds to somber echoes for
sculpted ears, fashioned in the style of your
own. You're an artist of flesh, perfection

built from emotion and blood that you meld
within as weight – your hidden canvas held.

(Bath Tub Message)

In the water, hot and quiet, you wait
unmoving for an internal motion.
Your feet are set steady and arms out straight,
floating. You stifle any vibration

of breathing, neck deep, as you stare beyond
your breasts to your silent belly watching
for the slightest sight of ripples. This bond
of water and skin, the subtle matching

of wombs, will let you see inside at last.
Suddenly, you feel a fret from within
then see the swell of gentle circles cast
and spreading in a path of echoes thin

and mute. Thoughtful and slow, sinking displaced,
you realize warmth has you both embraced.

(The Idea Alone)

"Everyone is beginning to notice
that there's another person in the room,"
you say, steadying your changing aplomb,
fishing bobby pins from your hair. "It's nice,

but people I hardly know think they can
touch my belly without asking." You bite
the pins, once pulled, between your teeth, the tight
twists behind your head spreading loose to span

your shoulders, each strand still moist from your bath.
"I humor them, but that's so personal.
They're stealing from me like some casual
shoplifter." Your hand slides a guarding path

down your cradle as you envision scenes
of protecting your child by any means.

(Idol Worship)

Your body moves more than ever below
the fall and lift of my hand in the climbs
and crevasses of you unfolding. Low
bends of stretching skin curve you along limbs

furrowing across the bed. This gesture,
unconscious and innate, has been lifetimes
admired – an outside view of a sculpture
fashioning inside you. These are the chimes

of perpetuation, steady heartbeats
resonating in harmony to call
a constant admission of fate. In sheets,
your draped ritual robes, I darkly crawl,

humming hymns upwards to your slim retreat
and, in devotion, kiss your holy feet.

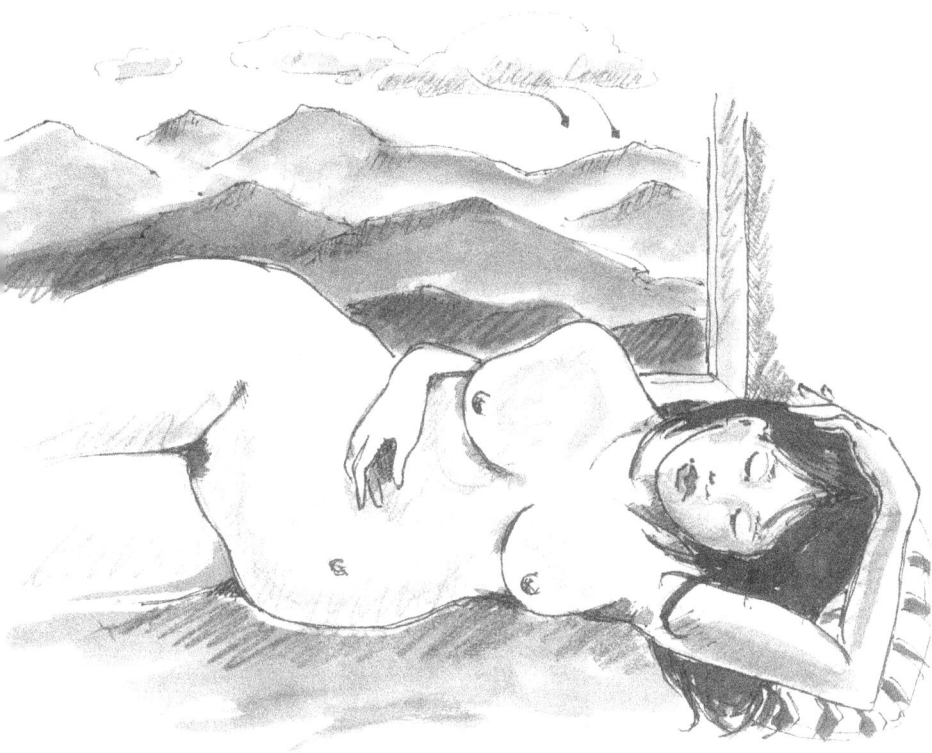

(Fifth Dream)

Knees high in the air, you stare at the masked
man between your legs. You're feeling no pain
as he issues pushes. Water sounds rain
on tiled floor as the effort you've been tasked

feels completed. The masked man stalls when asked
by you to see the birth. With a certain
observant stare he surveys with disdain
what he holds from your sight. Then, you are basked

in the lit joy you delivered. He holds
a red balloon, gleaming slick, dotted with
white barnacles marrowed and intricate.

You smile as he places it on the folds
of your chest and you stroke the clammy pith
of its red skin, so smoothly delicate.

(Stretching Wakeup)

The small something inside subtly stirs
you to awareness, reaching around deep-
rooted dreams, steeping in fog-colored sleep.
You both have turned together so long, sure

of shared comfort and placement within bounds.
Now, this is a scribbling outside the lines,
beyond the sinew barrier confines
below sheets and skin. You swear you hear sounds

of liquid moving as the coil springs long
and defined, with formed joints testing limits.
It is a firmness pushing set permits
of a union shaped in growth. A new, strong

pressure wakes you to the ripening cast
discovering itself from your contrast.

Detail Three

By the end of the third trimester, the mother will have gained an average of twenty-five to thirty pounds, around seven and a half of that being the weight of the conceived, which is now about nineteen inches long. Fatigue returns along with a general feeling of discomfort from the weight gain effects on the mother's back and the compression of the internal organs. As the conceived descends, much of this pressure to the lungs and diaphragm are relieved in what is called "the lightening." Fetal movement is prevalent along with anxieties, apprehensions and impatience about the coming birth.

The mother's body continues its expansion, resulting in clumsiness and more visible stretch marks. Leg cramps can continue, as well as frequent urination, pelvic discomfort, difficulty sleeping, and a further increase in appetite.

The conceived moves limited in the decreasing space. It can open and close its eyes, its face appears like a newborn's, and, by the end of the trimester, its head is engaged in the pelvis, causing practice contractions that prepare the mother's body for delivery.

Third Trimester :
Preparation Day

(To a Mother Soon, Sleeping)

Your shape is paramount. The cushions hold
you lazily and are little help for
lending relief from the night's uncontrolled
turning to find that one position more

painless than the last. There are set limits
confining you to tight and rehearsed shifts
in a series of tense returns. It pits
your body against your sleep as the rifts

of dreams cross and fade into consciousness.
There is nothing level on either side
but grasps and gasps of shallow breathlessness
around stiff joints that nearly sound. Each tried

strategy amplifies your belly's press
as tiny kicks flick against the mattress.

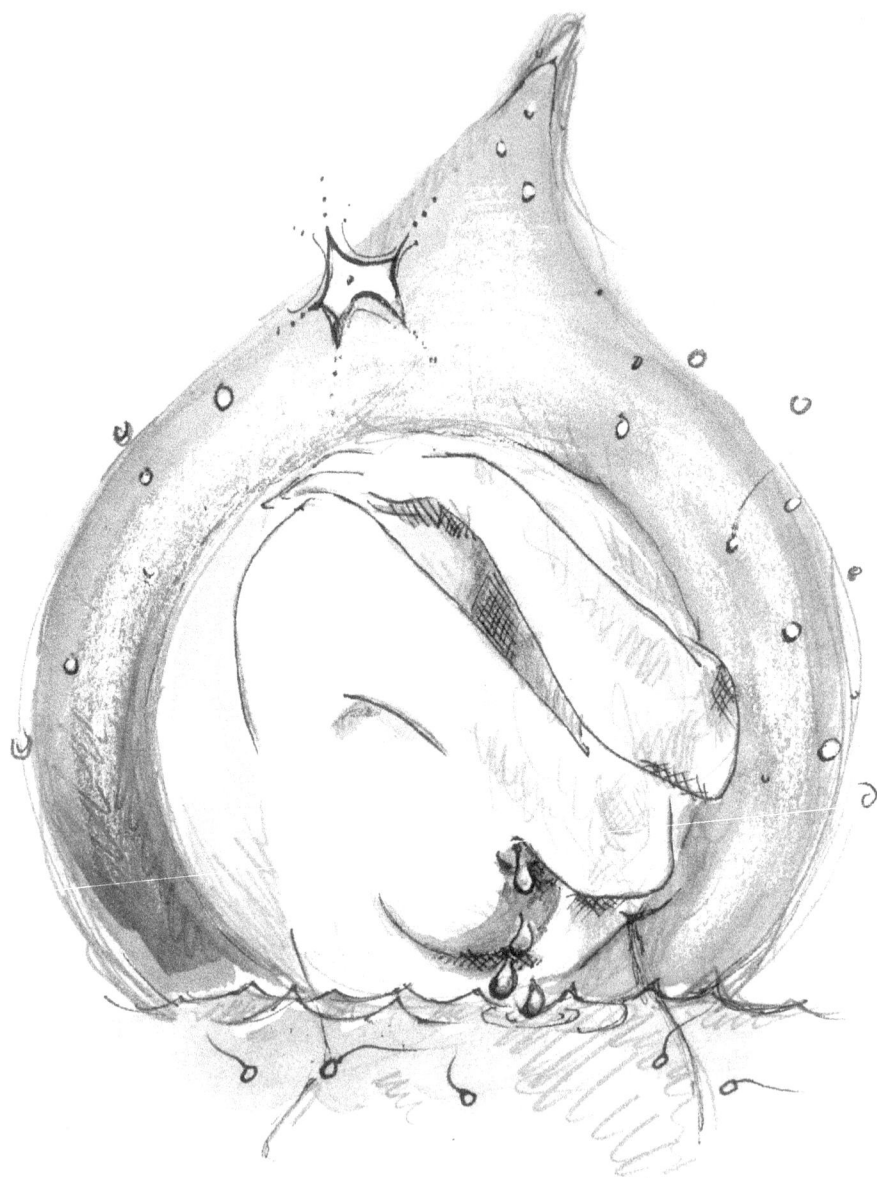

(Sixth Dream)

The baby rests in your arms as your rocks
in succession begin leading to sleep.
You wake to nuzzling at your breast, short peeps
of enfamined sounds. You lightly unlock

your bulging breast to issue the saved stock,
watery and skin-warm, trying to sweep
the child from comfort to comfort and keep
cries nearly unheard but a sudden shock

of milk overflows. Crying through bubbles,
the baby struggles. You have no control
as the strong stream coats the baby's features

and pools beneath you. The liquid marbles
solid white and your milk-stone baby rolls
to the floor – a wobbling silent sculpture.

(The Lightening)

Overnight, the built pressure unbuckles
and you wake with a deep breath forgotten
from months ago. The slide of your molten
binding lengthens your lungs and unwrinkles

creased trappings. The few inches of relief
feel miles deep compared with the shared space
once figured. This engagement is displaced
forward and low – the budding of a leaf

pushing freer. Yet this release runs nibs
of pain at the arch of your back, grinding
turns at your hinge with a corkscrew winding
nerves through your legs. A renewed view of ribs

reminds you of the waist you used to sway
that only waddles when you walk today.

(Weight, Etc.)

These new intricacies and additions,
both inside and around you, have tempered
each space compressed. Embodied in whimpered
sighs, standing on the scale, your condition

is weighed in full at its utmost extreme.
The numbers spin adding the four extra
pounds of blood and a one-pound placenta,
amniotic and other fluids seem

to make up six more, plus one for each breast,
two pounds of nurturing uterus weight,
with ten more pounds throughout to illustrate
what it takes to support your baby best,

who adds another some seven pounds alone,
as the scale stops and you miserably moan.

(A Number of Games)

The protrusion of a foot, a slight jut,
can be pinched with your fingertips to play
a mini tug-of-war. A simple strut
turns you to a swing and a tethered sway

swirls inside as jumps and rolls. You can smooth
your hand along your stomach's side to cause
a series of swift jabs trailing the soothe
of your touch. When you hum a song and pause

you will be bumped, prodded for an encore.
The most loved and practiced, the very best
example collaboration is sure,
takes one finger pointed and the simplest

of pokes to your belly's rind. It returns
a mimicked tap issuing your next turn.

(Seventh Dream – A Nap)

Crouching to a squat from cramps, you embrace
your knees and push through the steep forced pressure
massing. Your body gives no disclosure
to cessation of pain or taxing pace

as something rattles from you to the space
around your feet. You fall from your posture
to sit and stare at a mounded mixture
of dust and dirt around a leaning vase

with a rag-doll enclosed. The button eyes
vacantly stare long with its shape compressed
to the bends at the waist of the thin glass,

one arm hanging over the ridge. Your shies
away turn to interest, watching its pressed
face warped against its crystal clear impasse.

(Tectonic Movements)

Exploring the globe of your midriff seems
topographical at times. There are plains,
smooth and curving, in a finely cast scheme
that rise without warning to wide mountain

ranges from an internal jolt. A heat
inside swirls to shape this new map structured
by your skin. The mountains sometimes retreat
to short hills that rove the plains and fracture

the glide of your hands. The external layer
is thin compared to the depth at the core
of the motion where, freely, the player
has its own bound upheavals to explore

in the movement that follows sensitive
touch on both sides of the sphere's perspective.

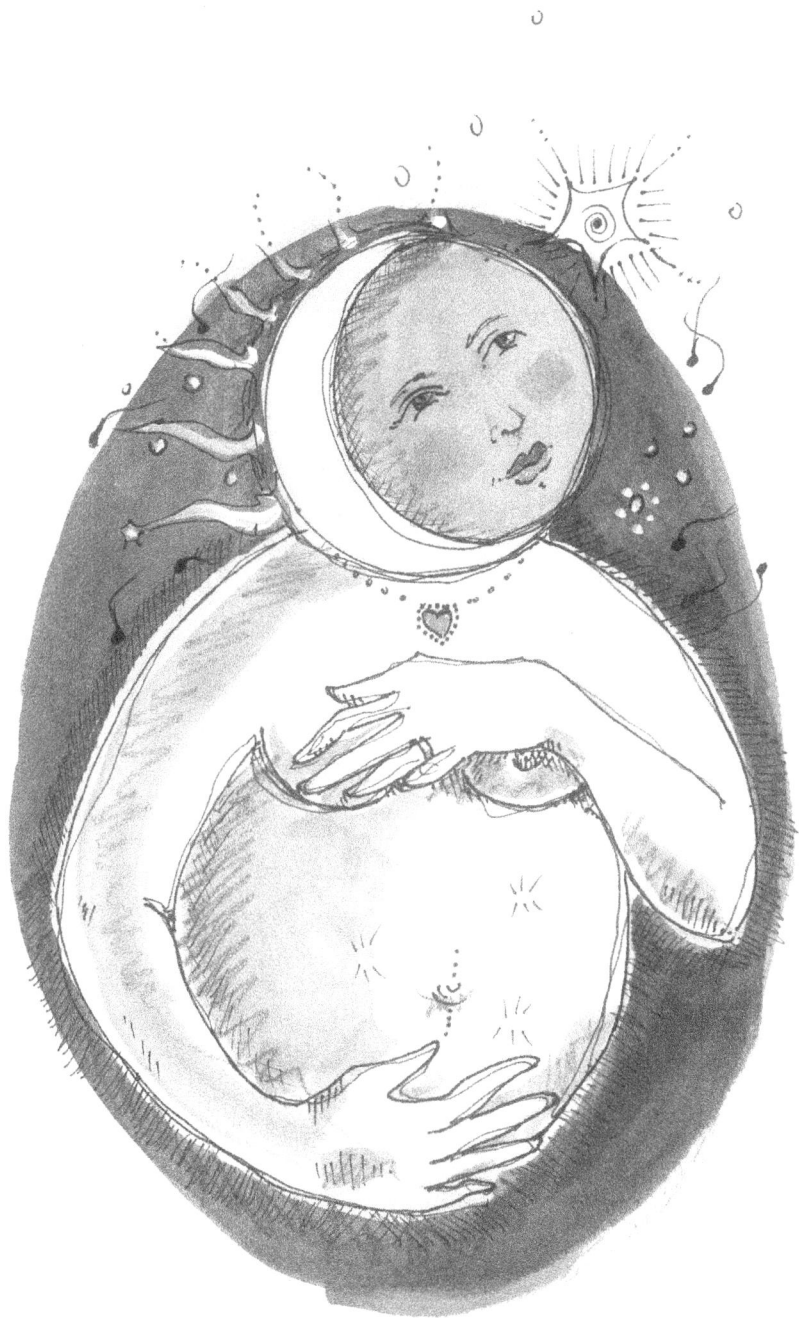

(The Skeleton Inside)

There is surely more to it than the sharp
elbows and knees that grind along sinews
and push momentary ruts in tissue
stretched tight, hip to hip, the fashion of harp

strings plucked. Another body, similar
to your own, is inches beneath your skin.
A compression of bones tempered as tin,
aged in rich liquid with the peculiar

glint of a laced shine. The head, chest and each
lanky limb has a bending resilience
to contract further to slip through the dense
plies of your layers. The tremble of its reach

is held and balled before you until forced
light gathers to lead down the plotted course.

(The Idea)

"It moves with me…with my breathing," you say,
"…with my belly." You cup its arching height,
blowing away a string of hair caught tight
to your lip. Your hands slide, pausing midway

down, holding the furthest reach. "It's so strange
to think I'm an opening to this world,
just walking around." The hair strand hangs curled
at your eye. Your hands glide to the deep range

of your hive – a flesh cornerstone. You stare
low and stand in shaped curves. "It's like a door
to a new place. A portal, waiting for
that one push, to lead here." The lone draped hair

flutters and your bodies lift in union
with breath, close now to that first division.

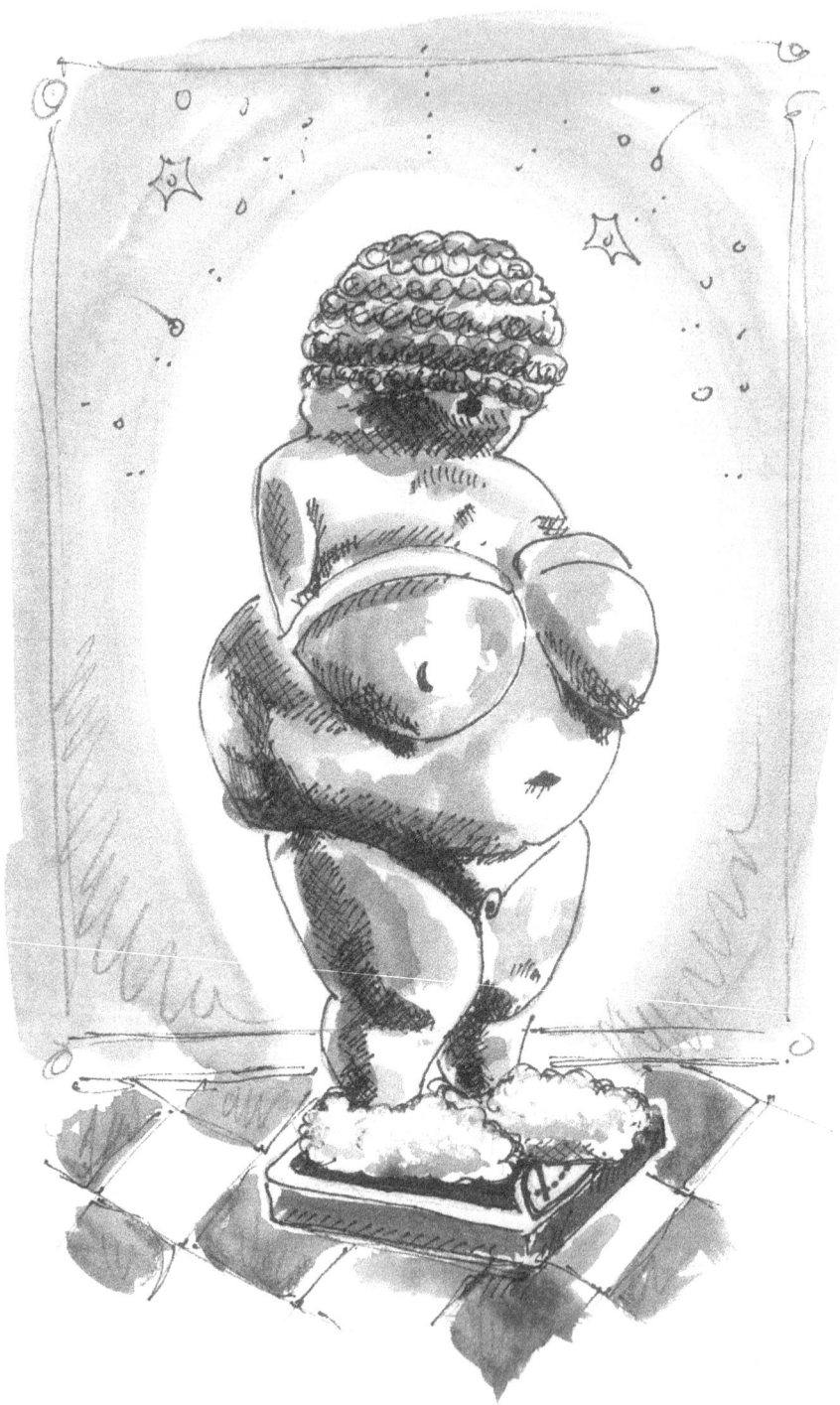

(Idol Worship)

The position is a perpetual
variable focused around a faint
percussion progression. A ritual
of taps in a steady pulse starts to paint

broad strokes, watery and blooming, along
your ridges and trim. It's never had such
resonance throughout – trembles that prolong
instances past instances. A warm touch

of breath leads the beat to timpani speed,
rolling over itself at a tumbling
pace, bulging peripheral views that lead
into the hazy summit. The climbing

lifts to air, and floats on a rapid hum
of moist skims to that final, deepest drum.

(Eighth Dream)

Standing in a fog, monks on swings whistle
by you, casting colored sand to the ground.
They quietly swing in long swells, the sound
of their scattering sand echoes. Thistle

width ropes string up boundless as they distill
serenity through specks. Patterns around
you shine as stained glass in each tightly wound
shape – a slow born beauty their epistle.

Between their steady swoops and flowing robes,
you rub the sides of your full-grown belly,
the prismed grains landing on your clothing

and hair. You don't brush them away and strobes
of light slip through fog, indescribably
enlightening you beyond rebirthing.

(Ready)

There is a sinking feeling in the pit
of your stomach. All the dreams are washing
away, assuring this fate. A dashing
pulse fills your veins and, as your conduit

season sifts in shifting layers, you begin
to revisit the list of sorted trusts.
The bags are packed in a checked-off fashion,
somewhat prepared, like you, for these quick thrusts

of compression leading soon to a flight
through the door. These heated spurs of riddling
aches are both the final nestling, tied tight
to you, and the final, closest cradling.

This odd coda of pain harshly issues
the separated bond that continues.

Epilogue

Falling Action

Adrenalin, ebbing to the corners
of your limbs, slows pace imperceptibly
to a lull in this supreme flash. Nimbly,
you catch fractured glimpses with a learner's

eye, memorizing and reciting each
lesson of curved and folded skin changing.
You hardly feel yourself rearranging
by the second while watching the spry reach

and twist of the variable immersed
in sight. The teacher illustrates with cries
and breaths in a tone that you recognize
as your own that has been some months rehearsed

in the waters of you. The song is ceased
as you two unite, finally released.

Fire Mobile
(the pregnancy sonnets)

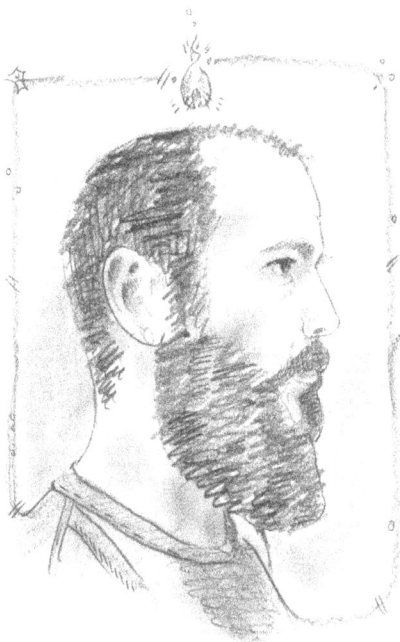

Matthew Porubsky is an internationally published poet. His first collection, *voyeur poems*, was awarded the 2006 Kansas Authors Club Nelson Poetry Book Award. He works as a switchman for the Union Pacific Railraod and lives in Topeka, Kansas with his wife and children.

Stella Robbins, artist by vocation and poet on the sly, does gallery work in oils, but gets much satisfaction out of drawing. She tries "not to let a day go by without putting down a line." A traveler by nature, Stella's work tends to be eclectic, with landscapes, animals and people given equal sway: a travelogue of life. These are her first illustrations for a book but she has done illustrations and publicity for community theater and drawings for children. Stella lives in Kansas.

www.ingramcontent.com/pod-product-compliance
Lightning Source LLC
Chambersburg PA
CBHW051736040426
42447CB00008B/1169